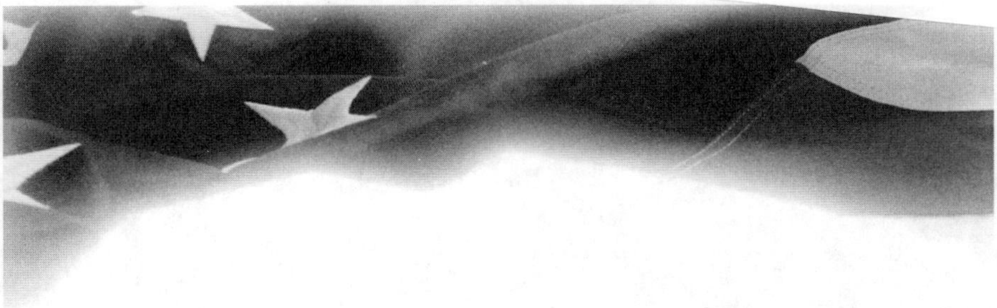

Aging in America

A Wake-Up Call and Call to Action for Seniors and Those Who Love and Serve Them

Linda L. Schlenker

A Perspective from one Healthcare Worker

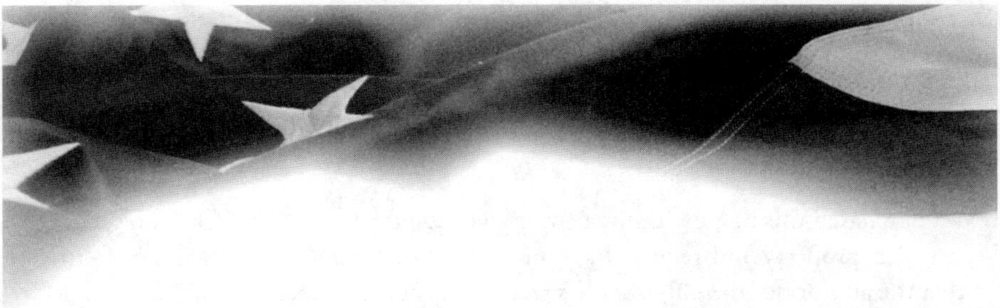

Aging in America

A Wake-Up Call and Call to Action for Seniors and Those Who Love and Serve Them

Published by: SIL Press

Visit our web site: www.safeandindependent.com

ISBN-13: 978-0-9795777-4-1
ISBN-10: 0-9795777-4-8

First Edition: November 2007

Also by Linda Schlenker...

How To Stay Safe and Independent in Your Home:
Fall Prevention for Seniors

Available in VHS and DVD
at Amazon.com

Dedication

This book is gratefully dedicated to

Brent, Emma, Matthew, and Grace Schlenker

and Mary Ellen Butler.

"America's health care system

is neither healthy, caring, nor a system."

– Walter Cronkite

Table of Contents

Foreword

As you read Linda Schlenker's insightful words, you may (as I did) hear echoes. The echoes are of phrases that most of us heard from our parents but shrugged off:

"A stitch in time saves nine!"

"Speak up!"

*"You can expect **only** what you inspect!"*

Through the thoughtful lens of a caring health professional, Linda gives us reason to reflect on those phrases and view them in a new light. She provides some realistic and sometimes disturbing views of the less-than-optimum state of health care in the U. S. The experiences she shares bring new clarity to our parents' almost forgotten words.

Linda's warnings are clear. Her words are profound. If ever we should heed them, the time is now!

Be proactive as you see to the needs of elderly parents.
... A stitch in time ...

Be a strong advocate for your parents.
... Speak up!

Be vigilant as you consider services and facilities for your parents.
... Inspect what you expect

Aging in America is indeed a wake up call for those who assist the elderly or act on their behalf. Linda's counterpoints to the bleak examples are hopeful and inspiring illustrations of "doing it right." May your experiences be included among the latter and contribute to reversing an alarming trend by focusing on quality and compassion.

– William F. Gillis
President
Parent Care, Inc.

Acknowledgments

I owe a special debt to Dr. William Stone and his wife, Maree, for their candor, support, and contributions to this project. I would like to thank Mr. William Gillis of Parent Care for allowing me to interview him and for sharing his priceless insights. I would also like to thank my book shepherd and publicist, Mona Gambetta of PCI Publishing Group and MRA :: PR, for believing in my message and guiding this project successfully from start to finish. Last, but certainly not least, I would like to express my gratitude to my dear husband, Brent, and my children, Emma, Matthew, and Grace whose patience and support made this book possible.

Preface

We who lived in concentration camps can remember the men who walked through the huts comforting others, giving away their last piece of bread. They may have been few in number, but they offer sufficient proof that everything can be taken from a man but one thing: the last of the human freedoms -- to choose one's attitude in any given set of circumstances, to choose one's own way.

– Viktor Frankl

On a recent Friday evening, my husband and I were having dinner at one of our favorite Phoenix restaurants. A gentleman, who appeared to be in his fifties, entered with his parents and was ushered by the hostess to a table near ours. The elderly parents were both using walkers and moving very cautiously. Just by looking, one could see they were both so pleased to be out to dinner with their son. Knowing my love of seniors, my husband smiled at me as I took in this heartwarming scene.

Witnessing this genuine caring was such a contrast to the week I had just endured. I had filled in at a nursing home where I had never worked before. Because they were particularly shorthanded and needed help, I agreed to go. It was, unfortunately, a horrible experience. Staff members were impatient and overworked. Most of the staff seemed to be either inexperienced or burned out. None of the staff members seemed to enjoy their job. I knew it was bad when residents thanked me for merely smiling! I felt a profound sorrow that these seniors had to endure this harsh treatment on a daily basis.

While working that day, I was stunned to hear a nurse suddenly scream, "Does anybody know CPR?" Of course the staff knew CPR! We were working in a healthcare facility where this was a requirement of all staff members. A patient at the facility had fallen to the floor and had no detectable pulse. Everyone was scrambling around in a panic—who was going to do CPR? Did this patient even want CPR? Despite the chaos, CPR was eventually started – regardless of whether she had even wanted it. Someone dialed 911, and soon the paramedics arrived and rushed her to an emergency room, where she eventually passed away. This episode was a fiasco from start to finish and an example of what happens when healthcare facilities are severely understaffed.

In contrast, here I was watching the elderly parents at the restaurant chatting about their week with their son. They looked to be enjoying themselves, a lovely sight to see. They scanned the menu and ordered a great bottle of red wine. This was a snapshot of what too many of us take for granted and too few seniors are able to enjoy: time with family, great food, engaging conversation.

As an Occupational Therapist, I have been dedicated to working with seniors in nursing homes, hospitals, hospice care, and in their own homes since 1989. I've written this book as a result of the helplessness and frustration I've felt watching our healthcare system deteriorating during that time: understaffed facilities, under-trained aides, poor living conditions for the elderly, elderly patients dying unnecessarily, confused and heartbroken families. Quality of care seems to be eroding at an alarming rate.

Witnessing the inability of healthcare workers to provide good care due to a failing system is frustrating, and the problem continues to grow. Those in positions to make change in our country need to be aware of the dire conditions that many seniors are living in and must be inspired to create necessary change.

I have included many of my favorite quotes in this book. Most of my favorites relate to working with ill seniors and many come from Mother Theresa. She had an amazing ability to speak the truth about caregiving in a clear, direct way. While researching her quotes for this project, I was struck by how much we Americans need her wisdom and how much our country would change if we took her advice to heart.

One particularly significant characteristic of Mother Theresa's work was her understanding of the power of touch, kindness, and a smile. She was always acutely aware of the importance of these things that we all can provide, and she wrote and spoke about this repeatedly in her work. These are among the things sorely lacking in our current system of healthcare, particularly with our seniors.

When illness strikes someone we love who's traveling down the road of aging, it can be devastating and overwhelming. Emotions run high and usually run the spectrum of fear, panic, anger, sadness, and more. Days are filled with doctor appointments, hospital visits, and co-pays.

In addition to the emotional costs, a health crisis taxes our time and money in ways we may have never anticipated. We quickly find that we must master a crash course in both patient advocacy and the business end of healthcare. Unfortunately, due to the immediacy of the moment, most learn by trial and error—often with painful and costly results.

This book is meant to assist seniors, their families, and the people who care for them. Information is critical when making choices about healthcare. Sometimes, the decision at hand is whether to move into an assisted living center or to age at home. When choosing assisted living, one must choose between multitudes of facilities or choose a private group home. If choosing to stay in one's own home, many need to hire an aide to assist them.

I hope what follows–as well as my experiences and education–will help you to make better informed decisions regarding future healthcare choices. Although healthcare has become a political hot button, this book is not meant to support any particular policy or take any political stand. This book is simply the result of my desire to share my healthcare experiences to provide insight for others.

"America's doctors, nurses, and medical researchers are the best in the world, but our health care system is broken."

– Mike Ferguson (R-NJ)
U.S. House of Representatives

1

Know Your Options

"Maybe in our own family we have somebody who is feeling lonely, who is feeling sick, who is feeling worried. Are we there? Let us know the poor in our own families first. We have old people: they are put in institutions and they are never visited; with less and less time even to smile at each other, with less and less time to be together. Love begins at home, if we can only make our own homes temples of love."

– Mother Theresa

Recently, my professional and personal lives converged. My beloved aunt, who was very ill, entered the hospital for surgery. The surgery had been planned in advance with her doctor. Her insurance company had also pre-approved the plan to transfer her to a respected rehabilitation unit of our choosing upon her release from the hospital.

Unfortunately, years earlier, she had made what we now believe to be a critical mistake. She assigned her Medicare coverage to an HMO. Because of this, a medical director at her HMO, someone who had never seen my aunt or treated her, was entitled to make the decision that my aunt did not need to go to a rehabilitation center once she left the hospital. Instead, the unseen medical director directed that she be sent to a nursing home.

Having worked in many of the nursing homes in our city, I was all too familiar with them. I could not allow her to be in any of the homes that were presented as options; I had witnessed firsthand the poor care their residents received. We opted, instead, to bring her home. What's important to note here is that I was not informed that she had insurance coverage for homecare. Until I asked about it, I wasn't aware that bringing her home and getting her in-home assistance was even an option.

I knew my aunt and her needs very well. More importantly, I knew where she would receive the best care. I had inside knowledge and did not have to take the word of someone else regarding the quality of care my aunt would supposedly receive in one of the suggested nursing homes. As a result, we made the choice to take care of her until she was well enough to resume living independently. Although the experience was still extremely stressful, I knew the available choices and which of them were not in my aunt's best interest. Her recovery went well. She will be ninety-six years old this year. She lives in her own apartment and needs assistance only with transportation and housecleaning. Because of my training, I was able to care for her. Most people, however, don't have my knowledge or expertise. Still, there is hope.

The most cost-effective choice–for the insurers–is usually presented to the family without their being aware that other options even exist.

Many of the families I have worked with over the years have expressed frustration in not knowing how to maneuver their way through the system. They don't know all of the available choices when making decisions related to elderly healthcare. The most cost-effective choice – for the insurers – is usually presented to the family without their being aware that other options even exist. When my aunt was denied her choice to go to a rehabilitation center, we were not informed that her coverage included homecare or care in a private group home. I only knew this because I worked in the field and was able to draw from my experience. Unfortunately, not everyone knows all their options and too often their loved one ends up in a less-than-ideal setting.

Ask questions until you know what all of your options are. And don't assume you'll be given the full range of options voluntarily.

Many times, people feel forced to make extremely important and life-altering decisions very quickly. They lack experience in making such choices, know little about available options and, worse, are unaware of the possible repercussions. Often, they learn after the fact that a different choice would have been a better one.

Particularly with an HMO, it's important that we make our own decisions and not rely solely upon the options our HMO provides us. Many times, we are unaware of all the choices available. Unfortunately, the only advice we are often given is from someone who may have a financial motivation to steer us into one particular cost-effective direction. Ask questions until you know what all of your options are. Don't assume you'll be given the full range of options voluntarily. The more informed you are, the better choices you can make for your aging loved ones.

"The care of human life and happiness, and not their destruction, is the first and only object of a good government."

– Thomas Jefferson

2

A Look Inside Nursing Homes

"We can never know how much good a simple smile can do."

– Mother Theresa

Our healthcare system in America is in crisis. We have a tremendous shortage of nurses, and it is no wonder. Most nurses are forced to work in settings where they are expected to care for too many patients. In most facilities, they can't possibly provide the quality care they would like to provide. Because of this personnel shortage, some facilities are forced to hire poorly trained nurses and aides, which exacerbates the problem.

As many who have visited nursing homes know, they are not always the types of places we envision our loved ones spending their last days. The odor can be stifling. Worse, it is not uncommon to find a nursing home filled with seniors lining the hallways, slumped in wheelchairs, sometimes moaning and pleading for help from a passerby. This seems to be a pitiful reflection of how far we, as a culture, have strayed from respecting our seniors, valuing their life experiences and the wisdom they possess.

Too many assisted living centers, care centers, and nursing homes are places I would never allow a loved one to enter. Most wouldn't either if they knew what the facilities were really like. However, families who schedule facility tours and interviews when considering placing a parent or grandparent, do not see that side. Prospective clients are usually given a grand tour of the area with the most active and healthy seniors. Prospective residents are often made all sorts of promises, including that they will be well cared for and loved. Most facilities will make promises of a nurturing, active, and attentive environment. Families must learn to get behind the scenes in order to see the truth.

Too many assisted living centers, care centers, and nursing homes are places I would never allow a loved one to enter.

My experience is that most facilities provide something very different than what families are looking for when needing to place a loved one. An unacceptable, but common experience, is an understaffed facility with too few nurses and staff to meet the needs of those they serve.

Nurses and aides are usually expected to care for far too many patients per shift. The result? Neglect. I can probably count on one hand the patients I've worked with in the last ten years who say they made the right decision to move to the nursing home.

Seniors left in these environments can become depressed and feel abandoned by the family who moved them there. Most seniors that I've worked with in nursing homes are lonely, isolated, and sedentary despite the promises made to keep them active. The majority of seniors that I've worked with wish to spend their final years seeing family and would like to be comforted by the closeness of their loved ones.

One of the most common reasons a family chooses to move a loved one to a nursing home, in my experience, is because they are unable to provide the level of care that is needed. However, in many nursing homes, patient call lights go unanswered for thirty to forty-five minutes or more. Unanswered call lights can exacerbate problems.

When patients have waited too long for help, they will try to manage without assistance. That can be a formula for disaster.

When patients have waited too long for help, they will try to manage without assistance. That can be a formula for disaster. For example, a patient who needs help to reach the restroom might attempt to go unaided due to desperation. Frequently, this results in a fall with broken bones—or worse.

Other times, a patient may press a call button for assistance with a health problem, such as chest pain, vomiting, or breathing problems. Untimely assistance may result in a crisis that could have been avoided.

Understaffing can also result in bedding not being changed when needed. Lying in a soiled bed is most unpleasant. However, it can be a serious health issue for incontinent patients. I have seen patients who have been left unattended until their waste congealed and adhered to their skin. This can cause bedsores that become infected and won't heal. In addition, when one is prone to bedsores, they need to be repositioned every two hours. When they're unable to roll over on their own, patients are dependent on others. When the staff does not have time to assist patients, they do not get turned on time. Not being turned and repositioned regularly can cause a bedsore in a very short period of time.

Many patients are unable to feed themselves independently, either due to physical or cognitive impairments. When the nursing staff does not have adequate time to feed patients, it's common for meals to be delivered and left sitting on the hospital tray. It can go untouched for hours because no one took the time to set it up for the patient, wake the patient to tell him it was there, or feed the patient. This is very serious, in particular for patients who are struggling with nutritional problems, weight loss, or diabetes.

Many of the aides are required only to attend a very brief class and take a simple test to become a "certified nursing assistant."

I've seen many patients injured due to inexperienced and unsupervised nursing aides.

It is not uncommon for nurses to be so overworked, understaffed, and under-trained that patient medications are delivered late or irregularly. This can cause severe repercussions. Improperly administered medications can be even more problematic if the patient does not have the proper food in their system.

In addition, if the patient gets their medication late for one dose, but then at the proper time for their next dose, they can have excess medication in their system, risking an overdose.

I have seen increasing numbers of under-trained staff members at these facilities. Many of the aides are required only to attend a very brief class and take a simple test to become a "certified nursing assistant." Many nursing aides that I have worked with are completely unfamiliar with diabetes, hip precautions, how to assist a patient getting up and down, and how to use common equipment. I've seen many patients injured due to inexperienced and unsupervised nursing aides.

On one occasion, I was sent to do a fall prevention assessment on a woman who had fallen and broken her hip. She'd had surgery for a total hip replacement following her fall and was sent to a nursing home for therapy and to assure her independence upon her return home. As with anyone who has had a total hip replacement, she was not to bend at the hips more than ninety degrees.

When I arrived to do the assessment, the nursing aide had the patient in the shower, sitting on a shower chair on its lowest setting, her hips bent far beyond the safe position. The aide had been trained that when someone is bathed after a hip replacement, she should make sure they are on a shower chair. My belief is that the aide was not doing this out of lack of care, but was missing critical information. She was not aware that the shower chair was not only to allow the patient to sit while bathing, but also because the patient needs a higher seat to avoid damage to her recently replaced hip. It was a simple case of not enough training and not enough experience that very easily could have sent this patient back in for surgery.

It was a simple case of not enough training and not enough experience that very easily could have sent this patient back in for surgery.

In an unrelated case, an attorney contacted me and requested I review the medical records of a woman who was injured in a nursing home. Unfortunately, she passed away from her injuries. As I recall, she was a relatively young woman who was disabled enough that she needed a Hoyer lift to get in and out of her wheelchair. A Hoyer lift is a device with a sling, which is draped underneath the person needing assistance. The sling can then be lifted up and down after being hooked into a stable frame, allowing a patient to be transferred to or from a bed or wheelchair safely.

The nursing aide assisting this woman attempted to get her out of bed with the Hoyer lift. The aide had never used a Hoyer lift and had not been properly trained to do so. She did not hook the sling into the frame properly, dropping the woman onto the floor. This aide, it turns out, had lied about her credentials and had not passed her certification exam. Yet, she had been employed to provide care. Her quote on the incident report explaining her attempt to move the patient – with equipment she didn't know how to use – was simply, "It didn't look that hard to do."

It's absolutely critical that when you choose a nursing home or any other type of facility for your loved one, you first familiarize yourself with it as much as possible. This means not simply relying on information you're given in a guided tour, but instead exploring the facility and talking to patients and staff members.

"But the greatest suffering is being lonely, feeling unloved, having no one. I have come more and more to realize that it is being unwanted that is the worst disease that any human being can ever experience. "

– Mother Theresa

3

The Choice to Age at Home

"Some 70% of seniors spend the rest of their life in the place where they celebrated their 65th birthday." [1]

Many assisted living facilities will say that they offer seniors more opportunities to socialize, and many have activity calendars filled with bingo and outings. It is my experience, however, that most seniors voice a desire to spend more time with family, friends, worship activities, and loved ones.

It is my opinion that if a senior can safely remain at home, he or she is much better off there. Research studies support that people are more likely to fall, more likely to report loneliness, and become more confused when moved to a nursing home. [2, 3] In the ideal scenario, one would remain at home with the support of family nearby. Many times, it is helpful or necessary to hire help for chores, but the investment is well worth it.

Seniors and their families need to clearly communicate what they want and what is important to them. Responses to these issues can help people decide where to live.

It is my opinion that if a senior can safely remain at home, he or she is much better off there. Research studies support that people are more likely to fall, more likely to report loneliness, and become more confused when moved to a nursing home.

When my aunt gave up driving ten years ago, we all knew that her current living situation would no longer work. I asked her a multitude of questions about what she needed. She told me that safety, security, and health were important to her.

She mostly wanted to spend time with her grandchildren, read, and attend church activities. We found her an apartment near us and next door to her church. It is in a gated community, so she feels safe and secure. She has housekeeping help, but does her own cooking and laundry. She rides a scooter to church each day and enjoys her independence.

Every family needs to communicate to find what will work best for their individual needs.

If a senior stays home, it may also be helpful to find activities to get them out of the house and with people, whether it's going to the grocery store, a place of worship, or visiting old friends.

One concern of a senior staying at home independently is that he may fall and not be able to get help for an injury in a timely fashion. Seniors may be statistically less likely to fall at home. [4]

A senior may, however, be more likely to receive rapid help after a fall if they're in a nursing home because of the staff, residents, and visitors around to potentially witness the fall and provide assistance.

To address this risk, one thing I recommend for seniors who stay home is a **Personal Emergency Response System**. This is a waterproof alarm button that is worn either as a bracelet or a necklace and never has to be taken off, even in the shower. The alarm button also comes with a speaker that hooks into the phone line in the senior's home.

If a senior stays home, it may also be helpful to find activities to get them out of the house and with people, whether it's going to the grocery store, a place of worship, or visiting old friends.

If a senior falls, he can press the button for help. Once the button is pressed, someone from the alarm company will contact the senior through the speaker. If needed, the company will contact a family member or emergency services.

Between the bracelet and necklace style, I recommend the bracelet. The necklace has the potential for the button to slip behind the senior's neck during a fall, making it more difficult to reach the button if injured. Also, most people are used to wearing a watch, so having something on their wrist feels more natural, especially for men. I have found that the personal emergency response button gives family members great comfort, knowing that if their loved one needs help immediately, they have a means to summon it immediately.

When a senior chooses to stay in their home, another important thing to consider is having a **home safety evaluation**. It is helpful to have an Occupational

Therapist come into the home to make recommendations to help a senior stay as independent and as safe as possible. Professionals trained in fall prevention know the hazards to look for and are experienced in ways to prevent the most common falls. It is typical for an Occupational Therapist to rearrange the kitchen for accessibility, recommend grab bars, remove throw rugs, and recommend shower chairs and elevated toilet seats.

Be careful of inexperienced people who have invested in a private care home for purely financial reasons. I have seen people open group homes because they have heard they can be a profitable business.

If a senior cannot stay at home, one option to consider is a **private care home**. This can actually be a wonderful and caring setting, if it is done right.

There are many things to look for when choosing one and I've incuded a list of questions at the end of this book to help you in evaluating and choosing a private care home. I recommend looking for a home that is owned by people who understand healthcare and are invested in providing a quality service.

Be careful of inexperienced people who have invested in a private care home for purely financial reasons. I have seen people open group homes because they have heard they can be a profitable business. These inexperienced investors open several homes at a time, with too few and inexperienced caregivers because it's cheaper to do so. Often, these "investors" open as many homes as they can and have no time to supervise each home to ensure it is being properly run.

I have visited quality private care homes that are owned by people who only own two or three homes in a small area. Ideally, the owners will have experience in healthcare, such as nursing or social work, and they are motivated and invested in providing good care. They will typically only take in four to six seniors at a time and will try to ensure that they will all be a good match together.

It is imperative that the caregivers are attentive and friendly so the residents do not feel lonely and isolated.

One should look for cleanliness and the absence of odors, as well as proof that there are regular and healthy meals, drinks, and snacks provided. The owners should be adequately supervising the home and must be easily accessible. It is critical that all caregivers be experienced, compassionate, and well-trained.

"Very old people love to have somebody listen to them and let them talk, even if they have to tell the story of thirty years ago. To listen, when nobody else wants to listen, is a very beautiful thing."

– Mother Theresa

4

Real People: Their Stories and Experiences

"I can also show you that people from all walks of life agree that someone who is sick deserves, in principle, compassion and care. "

– Paul Farmer MD, PhD, Harvard Medical School

I would like to describe the experiences of a few families whom I have worked with in recent years. It was stories like these which moved me to write this book, sharing my experiences and theirs. Specifics have been changed to protect their privacy. Their stories, however, are both common and familiar.

The Devoted Daughter

"If anyone wants to help me, let them begin at home.
There is help needed on your doorstep. "
– Mother Theresa

About a year ago, I was asked to go visit a home to complete a fall prevention assessment. As is usually the case, the senior had already fallen a couple times and the family was quite interested in doing everything they could to prevent another fall.

Upon arrival, a warm, friendly woman greeted me at the door. She was full of humor and personality. She escorted me into a lovely home and introduced me to her father. He was on hospice care and was clearly quite ill. He was confined to a wheelchair and needed assistance to do everything: toileting, getting from a chair to his wheelchair, getting in and out of bed, meal preparation, etc. His daughter was mostly concerned about his ability to toilet and bathe without falling and with her ability to safely assist him. The family was in the process of remodeling the bathroom to accommodate him and needed specifics about how to proceed.

What really struck me about this particular case was that this daughter was not only caring for her dying father, but also for her mother who had dementia. Her mother needed just as much care as her father, if not more. A diagnosis of dementia can be very challenging for a caregiver. I very quickly realized what this dear daughter had taken on. She was living with her parents full-time and tending to all their needs in an extraordinary way. It was just the three of them in the home; I wondered how she was doing it and how she wasn't burnt out.

She explained that prior to moving in with her parents, she was living on her own on the other side of the country. She was not married, had no children, and had graduated from a prestigious university. She had worked hard on her career and was enjoying much success with it. Her father, however, had been becoming more ill and her mother more confused. Her other siblings lived in the same state as her parents, but did not seem to find time for them. Every time her father or mother had a crisis, this devoted daughter dropped everything and flew in from out of state. Many times, she said, she even beat her siblings to the hospital even though they lived in town.

On one of her last trips to manage a health crisis with her parents, her father took her aside and asked her to take care of them. He was concerned, not only for himself but also for his confused wife whom he knew may very well outlive him. No one else was as dedicated as this daughter. He knew what he was asking her to give up and he knew he had very little to offer her. She said she didn't even give it a second thought. She sold her home, took a break from her successful career, and became a full-time caregiver.

Now her days are filled with bathroom trips, making meals, doctor visits, and giving medications. She is also managing the revolving door for all of us health workers who continue to visit their home in hopes of offering something helpful, some way to give her and her parents a higher quality of life, respect, and dignity.

No one else was as dedicated as this daughter. He knew what he was asking her to give up and he knew he had very little to offer her.

I am sure I can't begin to realize the contrast between her life now and what it had been: business suits, lunches out with friends, vacations in beautiful places, and a good night's sleep. When I point this out to her, she smiles and reminds me that this time is very short and this is all she has left with them. As I was leaving after my last visit there, I looked back to see her parents sitting in "his and hers" matching recliner chairs in front of the television set. They were holding hands and singing, "Take Me Out to the Ball Game."

Many Regrets

"Indifference and neglect often do much more damage than outright dislike."
– J.K. Rowling

Because of my extensive experience in fall prevention, I have been asked by attorneys on numerous occasions to review medical records of someone who was injured in a nursing home. They want my opinion about whether it was an unavoidable accident or something that should have been prevented. Unfortunately, they can be heartbreaking cases of families making the best decisions they can under very stressful circumstances. They trust that the professionals in the assisted living center they choose will take care of their loved one—and they have been failed miserably.

One family was very worried about their father who was living with them in a guest quarters on their property. He had been frequently dizzy and had fallen a number of times. One night in particular, he had gotten up to go to the bathroom and had fallen and hit his head. The family rushed him to the hospital for treatment.

Families trust that the professionals in the assisted living center they choose will take care of their loved one—and they have been failed miserably.

After many hours in the emergency room, he was admitted for dehydration and low blood pressure. He spent a day or two in the hospital, then the hospital staff told the family that they needed to put him in a nursing center to get stronger.

They said he would receive physical and occupational therapy to help him regain his strength and become more independent. They told the family it wasn't safe for him to go home and that the nursing center was actually the loving, best choice for their father.

The family hesitated at the thought of putting him in a nursing home, but reluctantly agreed. The family was told by these professionals that it was best for him. The father wasn't in the nursing home forty-eight hours when he got up, unsupervised, to go to the bathroom. He fell again on his way to the toilet and died from the injuries.

The family felt guilty about their decision, yet they were not given any alternatives and they were unaware of any other options. They were not told about home care options or about private homes that accept seniors and provide around-the-clock care and therapy services. They were making inexperienced decisions under stressful circumstances and believed the advice of people who were probably making financially-based decisions.

Many families find themselves making inexperienced decisions under stressful circumstances and believed the advice of people who were probably making financially-based decisions.

The Frustrated Son

"You must not lose faith in humanity. Humanity is an ocean; if a few drops of the ocean are dirty, the ocean does not become dirty. "
– Mohandas Gandhi

A nursing home in my area was very busy and needed an Occupational Therapist to assist with some patients. I was asked to help and agreed to go. While I was there, I was sitting at the nurse's station reviewing a chart of a patient I was going to see. I noticed a man standing at the nurse's station trying to get someone's attention. There were many people standing around, but nobody was helping him. I was completely unfamiliar with the place, but could see he needed assistance. I asked him if there was something I could do for him.

He explained that his mother had been a patient there and he had come for her medical records. I found someone to help him and was deeply moved to hear his story. He was very distraught at the care his mother received while she was there. He lived out of state and had been in town to visit his mother. He could tell she wasn't feeling well and was in distress. He told everyone at the nursing home who would listen to him that his mother needed help, and he pleaded for someone to find out what was going on with her.

I wanted him to know that although I didn't know him and I didn't work with his mother, I cared.

Apparently, his requests for attention and help were dismissed and he was told she was fine. Nothing was done until it was too late. At the time this gentleman came to pick up his mother's records, his mother was in critical condition at a nearby hospital, not expected to survive. It appeared the staff at the facility continued to dismiss her son and his concerns.

The pain on this man's face, the extreme grief, was a powerful thing to see. It was so apparent that he was absolutely heartbroken. This young, tall, fit, beautiful man had been brought to his knees. He had entrusted his mother to people who failed her and now were treating him with complete apathy.

It stayed with me for a long, long time and disturbed me greatly. I wanted him to know that someone in the field of senior healthcare did care. I wanted him to know that although I didn't know him or his mother, I cared.

Later that day, he called my employer and asked to speak with me. He had noticed my name and my company's name on my name badge and had tracked down the company number. When we spoke, he thanked me for helping him. I was so grateful he called and was grateful to know that our connection made a difference. I felt at that time, and still do, responsibility for representing the healthcare industry in a compassionate manner.

> We as healthcare workers need to listen more to families, to those who know our patients better than we ever could.
>
> The reality is that the family may very well notice something before we do because they know the patient so well.

It was a tremendous learning experience to realize that very small gestures during times of intense emotion can truly make a difference. I really didn't do anything for this man other than show I cared. That day was also a powerful reminder that we as healthcare workers need to listen more to families, to those who know our patients better than we ever could. It appears common for people who are constantly working with debilitated people and their worried families to stop taking family concerns seriously, particularly when healthcare workers are functioning under very difficult and stressful circumstances. The reality is the family is likely to notice something before we do because they know the patient. It is much better to listen to a family member's worries than to wish we had later.

Finding the Right Fit

"Old age, believe me, is a good and pleasant thing.
It is true you are gently shouldered off the stage, but then you are given
such a comfortable front stall as spectator. "
– Confucius

During another fall prevention visit, I had the opportunity to meet a lovely lady in her late seventies. She was widowed and living in a private care home. She was alert, but slightly confused. She needed a little supervision for bathing and dressing to avoid a fall and needed someone to make her meals for her. She also needed someone to manage her daily medications. I made a few recommendations for fall prevention, but all in all, the care home was doing everything right. There were no throw rugs, she had grab bars in all the right places, and an elevated toilet seat and shower chair had been installed.

I learned she had family in the area. Her children were married, with kids and grandkids. They were all working and had busy lives. They spent a great deal of time with this senior and always included her in weekend activities, holidays, and family meals. They loved her very much, but worried that they couldn't provide her the assistance she needed in their homes and felt she wasn't safe in her own. They searched high and low and found this lovely private care home near them.

One family searched high and low and found this lovely private care home near them.

The residents all appeared well cared for, and a number of qualified nursing assistants were there twenty-four hours a day. This family found a solution that worked for all of them.

The care home looked like a private residence. It was clean, spacious, and handicapped accessible. It had no foul odor. On the contrary, the place smelled like a home-cooked meal was being prepared. Everyone there looked happy, including the patient I was seeing. A married couple owned the home—the husband is a social worker and the wife is a nurse. They opened this home in response to the horrors they saw in nursing homes. Each resident of their home had separate bedrooms, and they only accept a handful of seniors at a time. The residents all appeared well cared for, and a number of qualified nursing assistants were there twenty-four hours a day. This family found a solution that worked for all of them.

5

Who Is Doing It Well?

"A small body of determined spirits
fired by an unquenchable faith in their mission can alter the course of history."
– Mohandas Gandhis

It's important to point out that although insurance companies seem to be ruling healthcare, and medical decisions made by doctors are being overruled by people focused on corporate earnings, there are some who are focused on one thing: putting the needs of people first.

I have interviewed and researched a number of organizations that are renowned for providing quality, comprehensive care without cutting any corners. What's interesting is that most are run as nonprofit organizations. I have often wondered why if the nonprofits in healthcare can do what they do so incredibly well and with such passion and compassion, why is it that the rest of the country can't follow suit?

The Mayo Clinic

"Have you experienced the joy of loving? You can do that as doctors.
You have a beautiful opportunity when the sick come to you
with great trust and confidence not only to receive a few tablets from you
but to receive your tender love and care and especially
when you have to make a sacrifice to look after the poor. "
– Mother Theresa

It's important to point out that although insurance companies seem to be ruling healthcare, and medical decisions made by doctors are being overruled by people focused on corporate earnings, there are some who are focused on one thing: putting the needs of people first.

As a home healthcare worker, I have often worked with many patients who were just released from the local Mayo Clinic. I honestly can't remember anyone ever being displeased with the care they'd received. Many times, they will credit Mayo with saving their lives. One gentleman shared with me, "I was told I only had a few months to live. Then, I went to Mayo. That was ten years ago."

What makes Mayo different? To find out, I went to Mayo and sat down for a long conversation with Dr. William Stone, a vascular surgeon and Associate Professor of Surgery at Mayo Clinic in Scottsdale, Arizona. It is important to note that Dr. Stone's opinions are his, and not necessarily those of Mayo Clinic.

The first thing Dr. Stone did when we met was hand me a brochure about

Mayo Clinic. Printed in bold at the top was: *Mayo Clinic, Primary Value: The needs of the patient come first.* He simply said, "That says it all."

Although Mayo continues to function as a nonprofit, they do not cut corners on the care they provide, and they continue to offer free or discounted care to those who need it. The Mayo Clinic receives very generous donations, in part because of their exceptional quality care, to allow them to continue their mission of putting the patient above profits.

I asked Dr. Stone what the biggest changes were that he has seen in healthcare over the last fifteen years. The first thing he mentioned was the ever-growing role of insurance companies. The practice of medicine is now managed in large part by insurance companies and the emphasis is very often on profits over patients and patient care.

I have often wondered why if the nonprofits in healthcare can do what they do so incredibly well and with such passion and compassion, why is it that the rest of the country can't follow suit?

Unfortunately, the insurance companies do not necessarily share Mayo's primary value of putting the needs of the patient first. In addition, the insurance companies have a growing and massive influence on the treatments that patients receive as well as where they receive them.

Reimbursement for physicians has become a system of quantity over quality. Physicians are being paid for the number of patients they see, not necessarily the services, or even quality of services, they provide. Therefore, with physician reimbursement already being cut dramatically, one can see the motivation that physicians have in seeing more patients per day, but spending much less time with each individual.

Dr. Stone is on a salary. This allows him to spend more time with his patients and he is not penalized for seeing fewer patients. He does not get paid more for seeing more patients. He feels strongly that doctors should not get paid more to spend less time with their patients.

My next question for Dr. Stone was what his advice would be for someone who is aging in America.

What are the pitfalls in the medical system that someone needs to look out for? The first thing he advised was to find a physician who will take the time to sit down with you or your loved one and take a complete and thorough medical history. It has been my experience that when seniors and their families have time to discuss both questions *and* answers with a physician, all are prepared to make better choices.

He did acknowledge that this is very hard to find and may not even exist at all in the manner that it did in years past. He said that when physicians have enough time to do their job, they rarely make mistakes.

Dr. Stone encourages patients to be sure that their physicians are communicating with each other. He emphasized the importance of each doctor knowing what treatment the patient's other doctors are prescribing.

The people in charge of running the for-profit hospitals and insurance companies would have to take a dramatic cut in pay and would need to redirect funds to patient care.

At Mayo, this is accomplished by a technology-based system where one doctor can simply press a few buttons on the computer to find out everything about his or her patient: medical history, specialists' reports, medications, etc.

My last question of Dr. Stone was: Why can't the whole country run medicine like Mayo? He explained that most hospitals are owned and run by corporations who are in the healthcare business and are making a lot of money. A typical hospital CEO will make millions in salary and bonuses every year. A Mayo CEO will make only a fraction of that. The people in charge of running the for-profit hospitals and insurance companies would have to take a dramatic cut in pay and would need to redirect funds to patient care.

Dr. Stone felt that much is being wasted in medicine today, from corporate salaries to a dysfunctional system of doctors being paid to provide less care to more patients rather than providing good care to fewer patients. He did feel that the country would benefit from a nonprofit healthcare system, although we are very far from that happening today. Dr. Stone summed up the current state of medicine very well: "It's a business now. It's no longer about taking care of you."

The practice of medicine is now managed in large part by insurance companies. Unfortunately, the insurance companies do not necessarily share Mayo's primary value of putting the needs of the patient first.

Parent Care

"For me, an area of moral clarity is:
you're in front of someone who's suffering
and you have the tools at your disposal to alleviate that suffering
or even eradicate it, and you act."

– Paul Farmer, MD, PhD
Harvard Medical School

Over the last few years, I have had the pleasure of getting to know a gentleman by the name of William Gillis. He's an amazing man with a very impressive resume. He has been the CEO of subsidiaries of Motorola, US West, and Charles Schwab, and is credited for the introduction of VHS, VCR, and Schwab's online brokerage service. His business-sense brilliance has been noticed worldwide and he was named a "Businessman to Watch" by *Fortune* magazine. He has received a Congressional Citation and has been a White House advisor on the topic of the Internet.

"The single biggest concern should be: that the senior's environment is safe!"

Fortunately for those of us living and working in the area of caring for seniors, this compassionate man has now dedicated himself to the cause of caring for seniors.

Mr. Gillis and his wife, a nurse, became long-distance caregivers for their elderly parents twenty years ago and have now transferred that experience into an extremely valuable online service for others who find themselves in similar positions. His company is called Parent Care (www.parents-care.com).

People who are caring for seniors can subscribe to this inexpensive service tailored to their loved one's zip code. A subscriber will find endless amounts of relevant information in their senior's neighborhood—such as free local medical equipment loan closets for shower chairs and elevated toilet seats, free medicine, home safety checklists, long-term care information, helpful Internet links, and updated articles written by experts in all fields related to seniors. As it is written on the Parent Care home page, *We have solved the caregiver maze, so you won't have to. We help remove obstacles to older parents' safety and independence even if they're not local.*

"Regrettably, far too little is being done to attack the fourth leading cause of death among those aged sixty-five or older—adverse reactions to medications. Each year, more than two million senior citizens are hospitalized due to sickening interactions between drugs and supplements they take. Over 200,000 die as a result. There are several correctable contributors to this problem."

I had the opportunity to have a question-and-answer session with Mr. Gillis on the insight he could share with seniors who are aging in America, and I asked him similar questions that I asked of Dr. Stone. Following are Mr. Gillis's thoughts, observations, and advice.

Question: What are the biggest changes you have seen in the last twenty years in healthcare?

Mr. Gillis: *Of the many changes in healthcare over the last twenty years, two stand out as the biggest. First, the long overdue addition of a prescription medication benefit for Medicare recipients is a great leap forward. Although far from perfect, its introduction means that millions of seniors no longer have to do without life essentials such as food and fuel in order to buy the medicines they need.*

A second, although lesser known, breakthrough is also positively affecting the lives of millions of senior citizens. Having good vision is the foundation of so much that senior citizens do. From playing cards with friends, driving, reading the newspaper, and avoiding obstacles that could cause crippling falls—good vision is paramount. Yet, cataracts have caused many seniors to suffer poor vision that threatens their safety and independence. Thanks to Dr. Patricia Bath's development of a laser cataract removal surgery technique and a more recent technique called phacoemulsification, millions of seniors are enjoying a return to good vision. A recent change in Medicare rules has put this once too expensive surgery within reach of all senior citizens.

Question: What do you think are the biggest concerns that loved ones of seniors should have?

That the senior's environment is safe! It's well known that the vast majority of seniors wish to remain independent and in their own homes. I passionately believe that seniors' loved ones should not only be concerned that their parents' environment is safe, but also that the loved ones do all in their power to assure their parents' safety. Doing some little things like removing trip and fall hazards (e.g., throw rugs and broken/uneven steps) can make for major improvements in safety.

What needs to change?

A fundamental change that is required is that we shift from being reactive to proactive in assisting our senior citizens.

Question: What *isn't* working in the system?

Regrettably, far too little is being done to attack the fourth leading cause of death among those aged sixty-five or older—adverse reactions to medications. Each year, more than two million senior citizens are hospitalized due to sickening interactions between drugs and supplements they take. Over 200,000 die as a result. There are several correctable contributors to this problem.

First, testing by pharmaceutical companies during trials should include senior citizens. I was surprised to learn that the majority of drug-testing participants are forty-something males. They cannot be regarded as a good proxy for seniors who metabolize drugs at a much different rate than young healthy males.

A second easy step to take is to make a list of all medications a senior is taking and have a doctor or pharmacist review them for potential dangers. The list should include not only prescription medications but over-the-counter drugs and supplements as well.

Question: What *is* working?

The lack of regular oral/dental care has been an issue that affected senior citizens for years. Poor-fitting dentures and loss of teeth directly affects their nutrition. Worse, open cavities and abscesses directly contribute to serious illnesses and, potentially, death. Unfortunately, due to the costs involved, many senior citizens do not visit a dentist. Thanks to a program sponsored by the American Dental Association, this is changing. Through a program called Donated Dental Services, the oral health of seniors is improving nationwide. Individual dentists and dental schools are providing free dental care to seniors who cannot afford their services.

Question: Who is doing it *right*? What are they doing that is different?

Although this is not exactly a healthcare example in the strictest sense, it has a major impact on the health of senior citizens and their continued independence. The state of New Jersey is following a phrase we've heard all our lives, "An ounce of prevention is worth a ton of cure," to assist senior citizens. Instead of waiting until a senior has fallen and injured themselves, New Jersey provides safety upgrades for their homes (e.g., handrails) in advance. Knowing that many would rely on the state for expensive long-term care, New Jersey is being proactive—spend a little now to avoid spending a lot later. A tip of the hat to one state that "gets it" and, in the process, is helping senior citizens to remain safe and independent in their own homes.

Question: What needs to change?

A fundamental change that is required is that we shift from being reactive to proactive in assisting our senior citizens. Unwittingly, the Older Americans Act of 1965 has caused our mindset to be one of waiting until there is a crisis before helping our elders. The Act was termed "a social safety net" for senior citizens. While unintended, this "safety net" mentality became a guiding force for elderly programs and how the families of seniors address their needs. To underscore this, several research studies indicate that 30 percent of seniors' relatives believe the senior needs assistance but haven't offered to help. Until and unless we become more proactive, millions of seniors will prematurely lose their prized independence!

Question: What do seniors and their families need to watch out for in seeking care?

One of the biggest issues on my radar screen is that families be very careful and thoughtful in hiring in-home attendants. There are several reasons for my concern. The first has to do with the qualifications (or lack thereof) of attendants. Demand for in-home care services is growing far more quickly than the number of qualified in-home aides. Family members should ask direct questions to ensure that the person to whom they are entrusting seniors' care is qualified. What type of license/certification do they hold? What type of training have they received? Can they provide references? Do they have a valid driver's license? Did their agency conduct a criminal background check before they were hired? Is it available for review?

Having good vision is the foundation of so much that senior citizens do. From playing cards with friends, driving, reading the newspaper, and avoiding obstacles that could cause crippling falls—good vision is paramount.

The more thorough families are in asking caregivers and agencies direct questions, the less likely they are to get an unwelcome surprise later.

I encourage anyone who is caring for a senior, even if the senior lives nearby, to subscribe to this very valuable service (www.parents-care.com). Mr. Gillis and his company have an endless source of knowledge and the resources to assist seniors and their caregivers, as is well illustrated in what he shared during our question-and-answer session. The best thing that one can do to assist themselves or someone they love is to arm themselves with as much information as possible, and this is something Parent Care can offer people around the country for about a dime a day.

St. Anne's Home, Little Sisters of the Poor • San Francisco

"I don't want the work to become a business but to remain a work of love.
I want you to have that complete confidence that God won't let us down.
Take Him at His word and seek first the Kingdom of Heaven,
and all else will be added on.
Joy, peace, and unity are more important than money.
If God wants me to do something, He gives me the means."
– Mother Theresa

It is important to know that there are some excellent assisted living facilities. St. Anne's is one of them. This facility is by far the most fabulous place for seniors that I have seen. It is run by a Catholic order of religious women, The Little Sisters of the Poor, who still dress in the traditional habit. They are some of the most loving and compassionate people I have ever met. Just as important, they do the job of taking care of the elderly very, very well. They have been doing it since 1901.

The sisters provide hot meals and a variety of activities for low-income seniors. They care for the elderly poor, assisting them not just with meals, but also with bathing, dressing, grooming, and healthcare. They do all this while relying on benefactors for 54 percent of the income needed to meet their monthly costs. Amazingly, these nuns literally go out into the streets of San Francisco looking for handouts.

Their home is filled with happy residents who love it there and feel fortunate to be there. Indeed they should, as St. Anne's Home usually carries an extensive waiting list for residential rooms. The residents are treated with love, respect, and compassion in a way I have seen at very few other places.

The meals are homemade and delicious. Families who are visiting from outside the area or whose loved one is so critically ill that the family doesn't want to leave the property may stay in a visitor's room. The family members are treated as valued guests. Aesthetically, the home is beautiful with lovely furniture and wood floors. The outside of the building is surrounded with extensive, beautifully landscaped grounds.

I remember thinking that everyone should pass from this world with such love, care, and dignity.

While I was there, I witnessed a dying woman surrounded by sisters praying and singing beautiful hymns in Latin. I remember thinking that everyone should pass from this world with such love, care, and dignity. St. Anne's does not discriminate on the basis of race, national origin, age, sex, or handicap.

One of the sisters told me that before she joined the Little Sisters of the Poor, she was working in a nursing home. When she chose to bathe a woman who had an odor, she was made fun of by the other people she worked with. It wasn't this particular patient's day to get a bath, but she needed it. Attending to this patient's need made this sister-to-be a target of ridicule.

Jeanne Jugan is the woman who started the Little Sisters of the Poor. She is quoted with saying, "*Be kind, especially with the infirm. Love them well. Oh yes! Be kind. It is a great grace God is giving you. In serving the aged, it is He Himself whom you are serving.*"

I encourage anyone who works in the field of elder care to visit St. Anne's Home and watch the beautiful work these women are doing. We all have much to learn from them. They are not profiting from caring for others; they do their work on a shoestring budget, and they do what they do so well. I sincerely believe it is because they are working for the love of what they do and those whom they serve.

6

Where We Go from Here

"America's health care system is neither healthy, caring, nor a system."
— Walter Cronkite

I have covered a good deal of ground in this book–the good and the bad, as well as some of the ugly. The future of healthcare does, in my opinion, lie with each person: what they are willing to tolerate, what they are willing to accept... and what they are willing to do to advocate, lobby for and initiate change. Some may say, "It's hopeless! How can any one individual hope to make a difference? How can one voice be heard?" My message is one of hope... that we, together, can affect change, and faith that, collectively, we can be a strong force for change, even in the face of what may seem to be insurmountable odds. Believe, as I do, that learning more about the 'system,' exploring your options within it and how best you can work as a healthcare advocate for those you love and we take the first steps toward change. My mission is to create awareness... to share stories and experiences that will move you to do the same. Nothing will change until we are acutely aware of the problems and exhaust every avenue on our journey for quality health care that is both compassionate and responsible.

Recognize the difference: For-profit versus nonprofit facilities.

The first thing that needs to happen is we need to recognize that we are dealing with a healthcare system that is vastly different from what it was even ten years ago. It has become a highly competitive business. Unfortunately, for the majority of for-profit healthcare businesses, it is about profit. To push profits, many hospitals and nursing homes are staffed as minimally as possible with poor patient-to-staff ratios.

The first thing that needs to happen is we need to recognize that we are dealing with a healthcare system that is vastly different from what it was even ten years ago.

It has become a highly competitive business and, unfortunately, for the majority of for-profit healthcare businesses, it is about profit.

Because of the shortage of educated, trained, and experienced nurses and nursing aides, the staff that is there isn't always the most qualified. Executives of for-profit hospitals and insurance companies are making millions, patient care is being cut, and quality is eroding dramatically. Once we recognize this, we need to educate ourselves and make better-informed choices. As mentioned, there are many nonprofit companies in healthcare today and, in my experience, they are providing exceptional care with compassionate staff. They are not in it for the money and are doing the jobs for typically less salary because they love what they do. A friend who was very successful in medical sales once said to me, "If you aren't chasing the almighty dollar, stay away from the for-profit and business side of healthcare."

Increase quality of training required for healthcare workers.

In response to the shortage of healthcare workers, training programs have been developed all around the country for medical aides that allow a person to become trained for different healthcare positions in just a few weeks. The result of this is a supply of workers who lack experience and adequate training.

We cannot replace registered nurses and licensed practical nurses with aides who have completed a training program consisting of just a few weeks. Many of these healthcare workers are the eyes and ears of a facility. It is crucial that they are experienced in all areas of nursing, most importantly in how to spot problems.

In addition, I have found that the old fashioned notion of treating others the way you would like to be treated is sorely missing in how we treat our seniors today. Many people come to the field of healthcare with an inherent gift in this. It is hard, however, for anyone to be patient, compassionate, and kind when under a great deal of stress, as many nurses and aides are these days with the chronic understaffing at facilities. Regardless, there needs to be more training for those in the field of caring for the elderly and the ill in compassion and kindness. It is truly remarkable how much difference eye contact, patience, and a soft touch can make.

In addition to compassionate care, respect must be given to our seniors. I cringe when I am in a facility and a condescending aide who is clearly lacking in training and experience is talking to a senior as though he or she were a misbehaving child. We must return to the days when we had insight into the gifts that we can receive from the older members of our society. We may never return to the day when most seniors aged with multiple generations of their family living in one home. With many seniors aging in corporate-run facilities, they are not receiving the kind of love and devotion that can sometimes only come from a family member. It is a shame that kindness, respect, patience, and compassion must be taught. If we must, however, then requiring that training as part of working in any career related to healthcare, including the insurance industry, is where we need to start with repairing our badly damaged healthcare system.

Do the research and know your choice before a health crisis, when possible.

For all aspects of healthcare decisions, including in-home care, medical insurance plans, and assisted living, one must take the time and do the research to assure that they know what they are getting. Seniors and their loved ones need to know what their choices are. This may take some time and it is difficult to weed out who is giving you objective facts and who is just trying to sell you something.

If possible, it is best to do this before a healthcare crisis strikes because it is usually difficult or even impossible to have a clear head and sufficient time to do this during a crisis.

There are good nursing homes, group homes, and assisted living centers out there. There are caring, educated, and experienced healthcare workers. I recommend actually talking to the seniors who live in a facility that you are considering to find out what it's like. Talk to the families of the seniors who live in these places. Is their loved one happy? Do they feel isolated? Do they feel that the staff is well trained and caring? How is the food? It's easy to be influenced by attractive marketing campaigns or to be swayed by the employee whose job it is to attract new residents. Remember—it is wise to not necessarily believe everything from someone who has a personal financial gain riding on the decisions you make.

Make sure your loved one has communicated their healthcare wishes, and assign an advocate for the patient.

One thing I have found to be crucial for people making their way through the healthcare maze is to have at least one person to advocate for the patient. If the patient can also advocate for themselves, that's terrific. It is, however, helpful to have someone else, such as a family member or close friend, ready to take up the challenge if that becomes necessary. This is exactly why it's important to have an up-to-date medical power of attorney at all times.

A related item that everyone needs to take the time to do is make your wishes known to those closest to you, should you not be able to make decisions yourself. Media regarding issues of life support has publicized the consequences of not setting up legal documents, such as Advanced Directives, outlining one's wishes. There is more to it than that, however. When other topics have been discussed in advance it can be extremely helpful to loved ones. Some of these topics include: whether one wants to stay in their own home with assistance, which hospital and doctor they want, what health plan they have, whether or not they want life support, whether or not they want hospice care. Many people even pre-plan their funeral arrangements. Clear communication is absolutely critical so that we can make sure our loved one's desires are met.

Conclusion

For people who haven't needed medical care in ten to twenty years, understanding the current state of affairs can be confusing. Dr. Stone summed it up well, I thought. It is a business now, and understanding that helps with decision-making.

Once we realize that people are profiting from our need for healthcare, we then must accept that the advice we receive from those employed by for-profit hospitals and insurance companies may not be in our best interest. We need to learn to do the research on our own. We must advocate for ourselves and have a back-up advocate waiting in the wings, should we need them.

We, as a country, need to continue to reexamine our entire healthcare industry. We need to look at how we allow hospitals, insurance companies, pharmaceutical companies, nursing homes, and assisted living communities to be run. It is unacceptable that quality continues to slide and physicians no longer get to decide what care patients receive. Doctors and nurses are living frenetically paced days, trying to provide care while understaffed and with reduced budgets.

Physicians' costs continue to skyrocket due to malpractice insurance premiums, while their pay and reimbursement are reduced to a fraction of what they were years ago.

Corporate greed and million-dollar executive bonuses and salaries must not be at the expense of the health and the quality of care that patients receive. Healthcare should be the focus of the healthcare industry. We must return to a system where doctors are paid for quality not quantity, where nurses have time to provide the care that patients require, where the treating doctors are allowed to make the decisions about what their patients need. We need a compassionate and patient-focused, quality medical system again.

Call to Action

I'm often asked: What can I do today to help my parents better prepare for the decisions that are ahead – and for my own health and healthcare needs?

This is what I tell them: First, encourage loved ones to share their feelings, desires, and questions regarding their wishes for when they need more care or are in poor health. Help them put their wishes in writing. Make sure all legal documents are in place to assure you and your loved ones have the future and care you desire.

Next, ask questions related to anything you do not understand. Ask those same questions again and again, if necessary, until you understand the answers and all your options completely. This is the only way to make good and informed choices. Know exactly what coverage you have and make sure you have it in writing.

Communicate with your doctors. Make sure they know exactly what medications, including supplements and over the counter medications, that you are taking. Make sure they know all specialists you have seen. Make sure you sign a release for all your doctors to have permission to speak to each other and have copies of your records sent to all doctors.

We are in an age where we must advocate for our medical needs. Be a voice for yourself and your loved ones. Be persistent: the squeaky wheel is often the only wheel getting the grease in our current state of health care. If you are denied the treatment, medication, care, or test that your doctor feels you need, speak up.

The next course of action is to support and get involved in groups and organizations that are the collective voice for and advocate for seniors. Voice your concerns to your elected officials. Let our elected officials know that the direction healthcare is going is unacceptable and we need change.

With the first of the baby boomers retiring in 2008, healthcare and all of its ramifications will be a hot button in upcoming elections–and for the foreseeable future.

*"Resolve to be tender with the young, compassionate with the aged,
sympathetic with the striving,
and tolerant with the weak and the wrong.
Sometime in your life you will have been all of these."*

– Dr. Robert H. Goddard

Questions to Ask...

When Choosing an Assisted Living Facility

1. How many aides do you have for each resident?

2. If I have to push a call-button for help, how quickly will someone come?

3. Have you had any complaints against you in the last year? If so, how many? What were the complaints for?

4. Have you checked the qualifications of all of your employees? Have you done background checks on them?

5. How often do you raise your rent and by how much?

6. May I talk with some of your residents?

7. May I see your unit with your residents that need the most care?

Questions to Ask...

When Choosing a Home Health Care Aide

1. How much experience do you have?

2. What are your qualifications?

3. Have you ever been arrested?

4. How often do you typically call in sick or absent?

5. Will you cook/shop/clean as well as care for me?

6. May I complete a background check?

7. May I check with prior employers to verify all of the above information?

Questions to Ask...

When meeting with your doctor

1. Have you received all my medical records from all of my other doctors?

2. Are you aware of all of my current medications?

3. What are the possible side effects of my medications?

4. Is there a possibility that there will be an interaction between any of my medications?

5. If I am undergoing tests, what is the reason for them?

6. When should I return to see you?

7. Will you make sure I get any instructions you have for me in writing?

Questions to Ask...

The owners of a private group home

1. How many homes do you own and where are they are located?
   Do you have any background in healthcare?

2. Do you manage the home(s) or have you hired managers?

3. What is the training and experience of your staff?

4. What is your staff-to-resident ratio?

5. What types of meals and snacks do you serve?
   Do I need to provide my own snacks?

6. Do you offer transportation to doctor visits?

7. Will you raise my rent and, if so, how often?

8. What efforts have you made to prevent your residents from falling?

Home Safety Checklist

Bathroom

___ Install grab bars wherever needed.

___ Consider a locking, elevated toilet seat with hand rails.

___ Use a shower chair or a tub bench for bathing.

___ Pull up throw rugs.

___ Install non-slip surfaces in shower or tub and outside shower or tub.

___ Use a night-light.

Kitchen

___ Place frequently used dishes, utensils, and cups on countertop.

___ Use microwave instead of stove or range top whenever possible.

___ Purchase and/or store heavy items, such as milk and laundry detergent, in smaller and easier to manage containers.

___ Prepare food and meals from a seated position.

___ Keep items on most accessible shelf in refrigerator.

___ Avoid reaching into cabinets that are too high or too low.

Bedroom

___ Keep a phone and light next to bed.

___ Consider the use of a bedside commode for nighttime trips to the toilet.

___ Assure that the bed is not too high or too low, making it difficult to get off of.

General Household

___ Keep a cordless phone with you at all times with emergency numbers programmed in.

___ Keep walkways clear of clutter and electrical cords.

___ Consider the use of a Personal Emergency Response System.

___ Pull up floor rugs.

___ Use good lighting.

Bibliography

1. ***http://www.seniorresource.com/ageinpl.htm***
2. Rubenstein LZ, Josephson KR, Robbins AS. Falls in the nursing home. Annals of Internal Medicine 1994;121:442–51.
3. ***http://www.coag.uvic.ca/resources_research_snapshots_social_isolation.htm***
4. Rubenstein LZ, Josephson KR, Robbins AS. Falls in the nursing home. Annals of Internal Medicine 1994;121:442–51.

Resources

AARP – American Association of Retired Persons
1-888-OUR-AARP
www.aarp.org

Philips Lifeline
Personal Emergency Response System
1-800-380-3111
www.lifelinesys.com

St. Anne's Home
300 Lake Street
San Francisco, CA 94118-1397
(415)751-6510

Mayo Clinic
www.mayoclinic.org
Jacksonville, FL
(904) 953-2000
Rochester, MN
(507) 284-2511
Scottsdale, AZ
(480)301-8000

Medicare
www.medicare.gov
1-800-MEDICARE

ParentCare
www.parents-care.com

About the Author

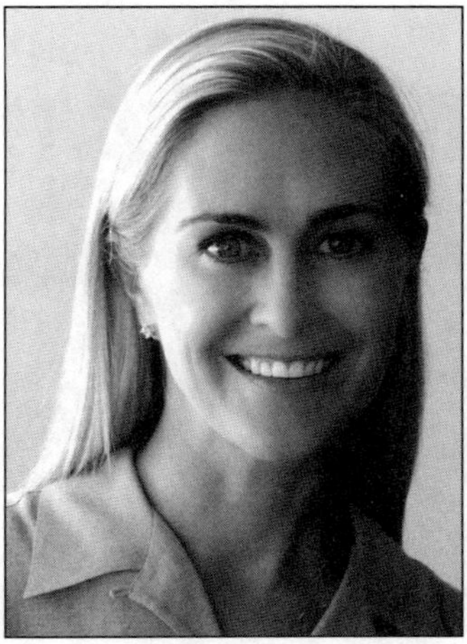

Linda Schlenker

Linda Schlenker is an Arizona-based licensed Occupational Therapist. She earned her undergraduate degree from Arizona State University and her master's degree in Occupational Therapy from Tufts University. In addition, she holds a master's degree in Counseling from Rivier College where she graduated with distinction. Linda has spent more than a decade assisting seniors and their families in many different settings: from private homes, to hospitals, nursing homes, assisted living, and hospice.

Notes

Notes

Notes

Safe and Independent Living

Linda Schlenker is a sought-after consultant and public speaker who addresses the challenges, obstacles and proactive solutions she shares in this book.

You can contact her at Linda@safeandindependent.com

Visit

safeandindependent.com

to learn more...

How To Stay Safe and Independent in Your Home: Fall Prevention for Seniors

Available in VHS and DVD at Amazon.com

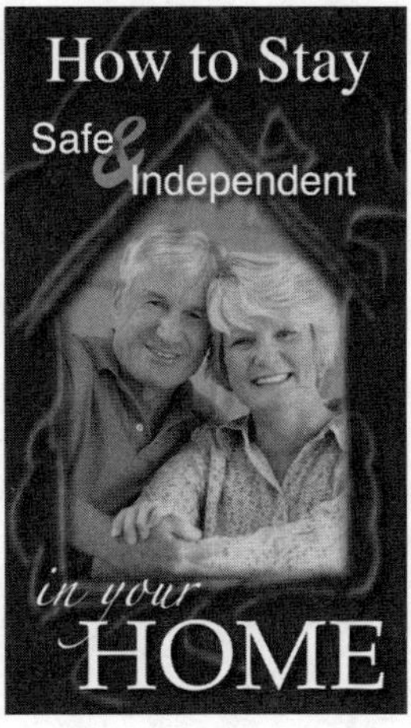

Stay Connected....

Receive Linda's monthly

Aging in America UPDATE

(It's free!)

Learn more at

www.safeandindependent.com